This journal belongs to

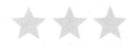

The 5 rules to create positive affirmations

- Always start with "I" or "My"

- Always use the present tense: say "I am" or "I feel" but not "I will" or "I should"

- Never use negations: say "I always succeed" and not "I never fail"

- Be precise and concise: don't say "I'm grateful" but "I'm grateful for having two awesome children"

- Always include a feeling

10 examples of positive affirmations

- My life is a joy filled with love, fun and friendship
- I'm a do-er : I take action and get things accomplished
- I finish every thing I start
- I'm responsible for everything happening in my life
- The universe provides for my every want and need
- I believe in my skills and abilities
- My body is a temple. I will keep my temple clean
- I make positive healthy choices
- I search for the good that comes even in bad situations
- I am so grateful for my life

Date

M ☐ T ☐ W ☐ T ☐ F ☐ S ☐ S ☐

One goal for today

Today's positive affirmation

My thoughts for today

My mood today

★ ★ ★ ★ ★ ★ ★ ★ ★ ★

Did I stay sober today?
YES ☐   NO ☐

Was today's goal accomplished?
YES ☐   NO ☐

What I am grateful for today

_____

_____

_____

_____

What I am proud of today

_____

_____

_____

My plans for tomorrow

_____

_____

_____

_____

Date

M ☐ T ☐ W ☐ T ☐ F ☐ S ☐ S ☐

One goal for today

Today's positive affirmation

My thoughts for today

My mood today

★ ★ ★ ★ ★ ★ ★ ★ ★ ★

Did I stay sober today?
YES ☐   NO ☐

Was today's goal accomplished?
YES ☐   NO ☐

What I am grateful for today

_____

_____

_____

_____

What I am proud of today

_____

_____

_____

My plans for tomorrow

_____

_____

_____

_____

Date

M ☐ T ☐ W ☐ T ☐ F ☐ S ☐ S ☐

One goal for today

Today's positive affirmation

My thoughts for today

My mood today

★ ★ ★ ★ ★ ★ ★ ★ ★ ★

Did I stay sober today?
YES ☐   NO ☐

Was today's goal accomplished?
YES ☐   NO ☐

What I am grateful for today

_____

_____

_____

What I am proud of today

_____

_____

_____

My plans for tomorrow

_____

_____

_____

Date

M ☐ T ☐ W ☐ T ☐ F ☐ S ☐ S ☐

One goal for today

Today's positive affirmation

My thoughts for today

My mood today

★ ★ ★ ★ ★ ★ ★ ★ ★ ★

Did I stay sober today?
YES ☐ NO ☐

Was today's goal accomplished?
YES ☐ NO ☐

What I am grateful for today

_____

_____

_____

_____

What I am proud of today

_____

_____

_____

My plans for tomorrow

_____

_____

_____

_____

Date _____

M ☐ T ☐ W ☐ T ☐ F ☐ S ☐ S ☐

One goal for today

_____

_____

Today's positive affirmation

_____

_____

_____

_____

My thoughts for today

_____

_____

_____

_____

_____

My mood today

★ ★ ★ ★ ★ ★ ★ ★ ★ ★

Did I stay sober today?
YES ☐   NO ☐

Was today's goal accomplished?
YES ☐   NO ☐

What I am grateful for today

_____

_____

_____

What I am proud of today

_____

_____

_____

My plans for tomorrow

_____

_____

_____

Date _____

M ☐ T ☐ W ☐ T ☐ F ☐ S ☐ S ☐

One goal for today

_____

_____

Today's positive affirmation

_____

_____

_____

_____

My thoughts for today

_____

_____

_____

_____

My mood today

★ ★ ★ ★ ★ ★ ★ ★ ★ ★

Did I stay sober today?
YES ☐   NO ☐
Was today's goal accomplished?
YES ☐   NO ☐
What I am grateful for today

_____

_____

_____

What I am proud of today

_____

_____

_____

My plans for tomorrow

_____

_____

_____

_____

Date _____

M ☐ T ☐ W ☐ T ☐ F ☐ S ☐ S ☐

One goal for today

_____

_____

Today's positive affirmation

_____

_____

_____

_____

My thoughts for today

_____

_____

_____

_____

_____

My mood today

★ ★ ★ ★ ★ ★ ★ ★ ★ ★

Did I stay sober today?
YES ☐   NO ☐

Was today's goal accomplished?
YES ☐   NO ☐

What I am grateful for today

_____

_____

_____

_____

What I am proud of today

_____

_____

_____

My plans for tomorrow

_____

_____

_____

_____

Date _____

M ☐ T ☐ W ☐ T ☐ F ☐ S ☐ S ☐

One goal for today

_____

_____

Today's positive affirmation

_____

_____

_____

_____

My thoughts for today

_____

_____

_____

_____

My mood today

★ ★ ★ ★ ★ ★ ★ ★ ★ ★

Did I stay sober today?
YES ☐   NO ☐

Was today's goal accomplished?
YES ☐   NO ☐

What I am grateful for today

_____

_____

_____

_____

What I am proud of today

_____

_____

_____

My plans for tomorrow

_____

_____

_____

_____

Date _____

M ☐ T ☐ W ☐ T ☐ F ☐ S ☐ S ☐

One goal for today

_____

_____

Today's positive affirmation

_____

_____

_____

_____

My thoughts for today

_____

_____

_____

_____

My mood today

★ ★ ★ ★ ★ ★ ★ ★ ★ ★

Did I stay sober today?
YES ☐   NO ☐

Was today's goal accomplished?
YES ☐   NO ☐

What I am grateful for today

_____

_____

_____

_____

What I am proud of today

_____

_____

_____

My plans for tomorrow

_____

_____

_____

_____

Date _____

M ☐ T ☐ W ☐ T ☐ F ☐ S ☐ S ☐

One goal for today

_____

_____

Today's positive affirmation

_____

_____

_____

_____

My thoughts for today

_____

_____

_____

_____

_____

My mood today

★ ★ ★ ★ ★ ★ ★ ★ ★ ★

Did I stay sober today?
YES ☐   NO ☐
Was today's goal accomplished?
YES ☐   NO ☐

What I am grateful for today

_____

_____

_____

_____

What I am proud of today

_____

_____

_____

_____

My plans for tomorrow

_____

_____

_____

_____

Date

M ☐ T ☐ W ☐ T ☐ F ☐ S ☐ S ☐

One goal for today

_____

_____

Today's positive affirmation

_____

_____

_____

_____

My thoughts for today

_____

_____

_____

_____

My mood today

★ ★ ★ ★ ★ ★ ★ ★ ★ ★

Did I stay sober today?
YES ☐   NO ☐
Was today's goal accomplished?
YES ☐   NO ☐
What I am grateful for today

_____

_____

_____

_____

What I am proud of today

_____

_____

_____

My plans for tomorrow

_____

_____

_____

_____

Date

M ☐ T ☐ W ☐ T ☐ F ☐ S ☐ S ☐

One goal for today

Today's positive affirmation

My thoughts for today

My mood today

★ ★ ★ ★ ★ ★ ★ ★ ★ ★

Did I stay sober today?
YES ☐　　NO ☐

Was today's goal accomplished?
YES ☐　　NO ☐

What I am grateful for today

_____

_____

_____

_____

What I am proud of today

_____

_____

_____

My plans for tomorrow

_____

_____

_____

_____

Date _____

M ☐   T ☐   W ☐   T ☐   F ☐   S ☐   S ☐

One goal for today

_____

_____

Today's positive affirmation

_____

_____

_____

_____

My thoughts for today

_____

_____

_____

_____

My mood today

★ ★ ★ ★ ★ ★ ★ ★ ★ ★

Did I stay sober today?
YES ☐　　NO ☐

Was today's goal accomplished?
YES ☐　　NO ☐

What I am grateful for today

_____

_____

_____

_____

What I am proud of today

_____

_____

_____

My plans for tomorrow

_____

_____

_____

_____

Date _____

M ☐ T ☐ W ☐ T ☐ F ☐ S ☐ S ☐

One goal for today

_____

_____

Today's positive affirmation

_____

_____

_____

_____

My thoughts for today

_____

_____

_____

_____

My mood today

★ ★ ★ ★ ★ ★ ★ ★ ★ ★

Did I stay sober today?
YES ☐   NO ☐

Was today's goal accomplished?
YES ☐   NO ☐

What I am grateful for today

_____

_____

_____

_____

What I am proud of today

_____

_____

_____

My plans for tomorrow

_____

_____

_____

_____

Date _____

M ☐ T ☐ W ☐ T ☐ F ☐ S ☐ S ☐

One goal for today

_____

_____

Today's positive affirmation

_____

_____

_____

_____

My thoughts for today

_____

_____

_____

_____

My mood today

★ ★ ★ ★ ★ ★ ★ ★ ★ ★

Did I stay sober today?
YES ☐   NO ☐
Was today's goal accomplished?
YES ☐   NO ☐
What I am grateful for today

_____

_____

_____

What I am proud of today

_____

_____

_____

My plans for tomorrow

_____

_____

_____

_____

Date _____

M ☐ T ☐ W ☐ T ☐ F ☐ S ☐ S ☐

One goal for today

_____

_____

Today's positive affirmation

_____

_____

_____

_____

My thoughts for today

_____

_____

_____

_____

_____

My mood today

★ ★ ★ ★ ★ ★ ★ ★ ★ ★

Did I stay sober today?
YES ☐   NO ☐

Was today's goal accomplished?
YES ☐   NO ☐

What I am grateful for today

_____

_____

_____

_____

What I am proud of today

_____

_____

_____

My plans for tomorrow

_____

_____

_____

_____

Date

M ☐ T ☐ W ☐ T ☐ F ☐ S ☐ S ☐

One goal for today

_____

_____

Today's positive affirmation

_____

_____

_____

_____

My thoughts for today

_____

_____

_____

_____

_____

My mood today

★ ★ ★ ★ ★ ★ ★ ★ ★ ★

Did I stay sober today?
YES ☐   NO ☐

Was today's goal accomplished?
YES ☐   NO ☐

What I am grateful for today

_____

_____

_____

_____

What I am proud of today

_____

_____

_____

_____

My plans for tomorrow

_____

_____

_____

_____

Date

M ☐ T ☐ W ☐ T ☐ F ☐ S ☐ S ☐

One goal for today

Today's positive affirmation

My thoughts for today

My mood today

★ ★ ★ ★ ★ ★ ★ ★ ★ ★

Did I stay sober today?
YES ☐   NO ☐
Was today's goal accomplished?
YES ☐   NO ☐
What I am grateful for today

_____

_____

_____

What I am proud of today

_____

_____

_____

My plans for tomorrow

_____

_____

_____

Date

M ☐ T ☐ W ☐ T ☐ F ☐ S ☐ S ☐

One goal for today

_____

_____

Today's positive affirmation

_____

_____

_____

My thoughts for today

_____

_____

_____

_____

My mood today

★ ★ ★ ★ ★ ★ ★ ★ ★ ★

Did I stay sober today?
YES ☐ NO ☐

Was today's goal accomplished?
YES ☐ NO ☐

What I am grateful for today

_____

_____

_____

What I am proud of today

_____

_____

_____

My plans for tomorrow

_____

_____

_____

Date _____

M ☐ T ☐ W ☐ T ☐ F ☐ S ☐ S ☐

One goal for today

_____

_____

Today's positive affirmation

_____

_____

_____

_____

My thoughts for today

_____

_____

_____

_____

My mood today

★ ★ ★ ★ ★ ★ ★ ★ ★ ★

Did I stay sober today?
YES ☐   NO ☐

Was today's goal accomplished?
YES ☐   NO ☐

What I am grateful for today

_____

_____

_____

What I am proud of today

_____

_____

_____

My plans for tomorrow

_____

_____

_____

Date _____

M ☐ T ☐ W ☐ T ☐ F ☐ S ☐ S ☐

One goal for today

_____

_____

Today's positive affirmation

_____

_____

_____

_____

My thoughts for today

_____

_____

_____

_____

_____

My mood today

★ ★ ★ ★ ★ ★ ★ ★ ★ ★

Did I stay sober today?

YES ☐　　NO ☐

Was today's goal accomplished?

YES ☐　　NO ☐

What I am grateful for today

_____

_____

_____

What I am proud of today

_____

_____

_____

My plans for tomorrow

_____

_____

_____

Date _____

M ☐ T ☐ W ☐ T ☐ F ☐ S ☐ S ☐

One goal for today

_____

_____

Today's positive affirmation

_____

_____

_____

_____

My thoughts for today

_____

_____

_____

_____

My mood today

★ ★ ★ ★ ★ ★ ★ ★ ★ ★

Did I stay sober today?
YES ☐   NO ☐

Was today's goal accomplished?
YES ☐   NO ☐

What I am grateful for today

_____

_____

_____

_____

What I am proud of today

_____

_____

_____

_____

My plans for tomorrow

_____

_____

_____

_____

Date _____

M ☐ T ☐ W ☐ T ☐ F ☐ S ☐ S ☐

One goal for today

_____

_____

Today's positive affirmation

_____

_____

_____

My thoughts for today

_____

_____

_____

_____

My mood today

★ ★ ★ ★ ★ ★ ★ ★ ★ ★

Did I stay sober today?
YES ☐　　NO ☐

Was today's goal accomplished?
YES ☐　　NO ☐

What I am grateful for today

_____

_____

_____

What I am proud of today

_____

_____

_____

My plans for tomorrow

_____

_____

_____

Date _____

M ☐ T ☐ W ☐ T ☐ F ☐ S ☐ S ☐

One goal for today

_____

_____

Today's positive affirmation

_____

_____

_____

My thoughts for today

_____

_____

_____

_____

My mood today

★ ★ ★ ★ ★ ★ ★ ★ ★ ★

Did I stay sober today?
YES ☐   NO ☐

Was today's goal accomplished?
YES ☐   NO ☐

What I am grateful for today

_____

_____

_____

What I am proud of today

_____

_____

My plans for tomorrow

_____

_____

_____

Date _____

M ☐ T ☐ W ☐ T ☐ F ☐ S ☐ S ☐

One goal for today

_____

_____

Today's positive affirmation

_____

_____

_____

My thoughts for today

_____

_____

_____

_____

My mood today

★ ★ ★ ★ ★ ★ ★ ★ ★ ★

Did I stay sober today?
YES ☐   NO ☐

Was today's goal accomplished?
YES ☐   NO ☐

What I am grateful for today

_____

_____

_____

_____

What I am proud of today

_____

_____

_____

My plans for tomorrow

_____

_____

_____

_____

Date _____

M ☐ T ☐ W ☐ T ☐ F ☐ S ☐ S ☐

One goal for today

_____

_____

Today's positive affirmation

_____

_____

_____

_____

My thoughts for today

_____

_____

_____

_____

My mood today

★ ★ ★ ★ ★ ★ ★ ★ ★ ★

Did I stay sober today?
YES ☐   NO ☐

Was today's goal accomplished?
YES ☐   NO ☐

What I am grateful for today

_____

_____

_____

_____

What I am proud of today

_____

_____

_____

My plans for tomorrow

_____

_____

_____

_____

Date

M ☐ T ☐ W ☐ T ☐ F ☐ S ☐ S ☐

One goal for today

Today's positive affirmation

My thoughts for today

My mood today

★ ★ ★ ★ ★ ★ ★ ★ ★ ★

Did I stay sober today?
YES ☐   NO ☐
Was today's goal accomplished?
YES ☐   NO ☐
What I am grateful for today

_____

_____

_____

_____

What I am proud of today

_____

_____

_____

_____

My plans for tomorrow

_____

_____

_____

_____

Date _____

M ☐ T ☐ W ☐ T ☐ F ☐ S ☐ S ☐

One goal for today

_____

_____

Today's positive affirmation

_____

_____

_____

My thoughts for today

_____

_____

_____

_____

My mood today

★ ★ ★ ★ ★ ★ ★ ★ ★ ★

Did I stay sober today?
YES ☐   NO ☐

Was today's goal accomplished?
YES ☐   NO ☐

What I am grateful for today

_____

_____

_____

_____

What I am proud of today

_____

_____

_____

My plans for tomorrow

_____

_____

_____

_____

Date

M ☐ T ☐ W ☐ T ☐ F ☐ S ☐ S ☐

One goal for today

_____

_____

Today's positive affirmation

_____

_____

_____

My thoughts for today

_____

_____

_____

_____

My mood today

★ ★ ★ ★ ★ ★ ★ ★ ★ ★

Did I stay sober today?
YES ☐   NO ☐

Was today's goal accomplished?
YES ☐   NO ☐

What I am grateful for today

_____

_____

_____

_____

What I am proud of today

_____

_____

_____

_____

My plans for tomorrow

_____

_____

_____

_____

Date _____

M ☐ T ☐ W ☐ T ☐ F ☐ S ☐ S ☐

One goal for today

_____

_____

Today's positive affirmation

_____

_____

_____

_____

My thoughts for today

_____

_____

_____

_____

_____

My mood today

★ ★ ★ ★ ★ ★ ★ ★ ★ ★

Did I stay sober today?

YES ☐   NO ☐

Was today's goal accomplished?

YES ☐   NO ☐

What I am grateful for today

_____

_____

_____

What I am proud of today

_____

_____

_____

My plans for tomorrow

_____

_____

_____

Date _____

M ☐ T ☐ W ☐ T ☐ F ☐ S ☐ S ☐

One goal for today

_____

_____

Today's positive affirmation

_____

_____

_____

_____

My thoughts for today

_____

_____

_____

_____

_____

My mood today

★ ★ ★ ★ ★ ★ ★ ★ ★ ★

Did I stay sober today?
YES ☐   NO ☐

Was today's goal accomplished?
YES ☐   NO ☐

What I am grateful for today

_____

_____

_____

_____

What I am proud of today

_____

_____

_____

_____

My plans for tomorrow

_____

_____

_____

_____

Date

M ☐ T ☐ W ☐ T ☐ F ☐ S ☐ S ☐

One goal for today

Today's positive affirmation

My thoughts for today

My mood today

★ ★ ★ ★ ★ ★ ★ ★ ★ ★

Did I stay sober today?
YES ☐   NO ☐

Was today's goal accomplished?
YES ☐   NO ☐

What I am grateful for today

_____

_____

_____

_____

What I am proud of today

_____

_____

_____

My plans for tomorrow

_____

_____

_____

_____

Date

M ☐ T ☐ W ☐ T ☐ F ☐ S ☐ S ☐

One goal for today

Today's positive affirmation

My thoughts for today

My mood today

★ ★ ★ ★ ★ ★ ★ ★ ★ ★

Did I stay sober today?
YES ☐   NO ☐

Was today's goal accomplished?
YES ☐   NO ☐

What I am grateful for today

_____

_____

_____

_____

What I am proud of today

_____

_____

_____

My plans for tomorrow

_____

_____

_____

_____

Date

M ☐ T ☐ W ☐ T ☐ F ☐ S ☐ S ☐

One goal for today

Today's positive affirmation

My thoughts for today

My mood today

★ ★ ★ ★ ★ ★ ★ ★ ★ ★

Did I stay sober today?
YES ☐   NO ☐

Was today's goal accomplished?
YES ☐   NO ☐

What I am grateful for today

_____

_____

_____

What I am proud of today

_____

_____

_____

My plans for tomorrow

_____

_____

_____

Date

M ☐ T ☐ W ☐ T ☐ F ☐ S ☐ S ☐

One goal for today

_____

_____

Today's positive affirmation

_____

_____

_____

_____

My thoughts for today

_____

_____

_____

_____

My mood today

★ ★ ★ ★ ★ ★ ★ ★ ★ ★

Did I stay sober today?
YES ☐   NO ☐
Was today's goal accomplished?
YES ☐   NO ☐
What I am grateful for today

_____

_____

_____

_____

What I am proud of today

_____

_____

_____

My plans for tomorrow

_____

_____

_____

_____

Date

M ☐ T ☐ W ☐ T ☐ F ☐ S ☐ S ☐

One goal for today

Today's positive affirmation

My thoughts for today

My mood today

★ ★ ★ ★ ★ ★ ★ ★ ★ ★

Did I stay sober today?

YES ☐   NO ☐

Was today's goal accomplished?

YES ☐   NO ☐

What I am grateful for today

_____

_____

_____

_____

What I am proud of today

_____

_____

_____

My plans for tomorrow

_____

_____

_____

_____

Date _____

M ☐ T ☐ W ☐ T ☐ F ☐ S ☐ S ☐

One goal for today

_____

_____

Today's positive affirmation

_____

_____

_____

_____

My thoughts for today

_____

_____

_____

_____

My mood today

★ ★ ★ ★ ★ ★ ★ ★ ★ ★

Did I stay sober today?
YES ☐   NO ☐

Was today's goal accomplished?
YES ☐   NO ☐

What I am grateful for today

_____

_____

_____

_____

What I am proud of today

_____

_____

_____

My plans for tomorrow

_____

_____

_____

_____

Date _____

M ☐ T ☐ W ☐ T ☐ F ☐ S ☐ S ☐

One goal for today

_____

_____

Today's positive affirmation

_____

_____

_____

My thoughts for today

_____

_____

_____

_____

My mood today

★ ★ ★ ★ ★ ★ ★ ★ ★ ★

Did I stay sober today?
YES ☐   NO ☐

Was today's goal accomplished?
YES ☐   NO ☐

What I am grateful for today

_____

_____

_____

_____

What I am proud of today

_____

_____

_____

_____

My plans for tomorrow

_____

_____

_____

_____

Date _____

M ☐ T ☐ W ☐ T ☐ F ☐ S ☐ S ☐

One goal for today

_____

_____

Today's positive affirmation

_____

_____

_____

_____

My thoughts for today

_____

_____

_____

_____

My mood today

★ ★ ★ ★ ★ ★ ★ ★ ★ ★

Did I stay sober today?
YES ☐   NO ☐

Was today's goal accomplished?
YES ☐   NO ☐

What I am grateful for today

_____

_____

_____

What I am proud of today

_____

_____

_____

My plans for tomorrow

_____

_____

_____

Date _____

M ☐ T ☐ W ☐ T ☐ F ☐ S ☐ S ☐

One goal for today

_____

_____

Today's positive affirmation

_____

_____

_____

_____

My thoughts for today

_____

_____

_____

_____

My mood today

★ ★ ★ ★ ★ ★ ★ ★ ★ ★

Did I stay sober today?
YES ☐   NO ☐

Was today's goal accomplished?
YES ☐   NO ☐

What I am grateful for today

_____

_____

_____

_____

What I am proud of today

_____

_____

_____

My plans for tomorrow

_____

_____

_____

_____

Date _____

M ☐ T ☐ W ☐ T ☐ F ☐ S ☐ S ☐

One goal for today

_____
_____

Today's positive affirmation

_____
_____
_____
_____

My thoughts for today

_____
_____
_____
_____

My mood today

★ ★ ★ ★ ★ ★ ★ ★ ★ ★

Did I stay sober today?
YES ☐   NO ☐

Was today's goal accomplished?
YES ☐   NO ☐

What I am grateful for today

What I am proud of today

My plans for tomorrow

Date

M ☐ T ☐ W ☐ T ☐ F ☐ S ☐ S ☐

One goal for today

Today's positive affirmation

My thoughts for today

My mood today

★ ★ ★ ★ ★ ★ ★ ★ ★ ★

Did I stay sober today?
YES ☐   NO ☐

Was today's goal accomplished?
YES ☐   NO ☐

What I am grateful for today

_____

_____

_____

_____

What I am proud of today

_____

_____

_____

My plans for tomorrow

_____

_____

_____

_____

Date _____

M ☐ T ☐ W ☐ T ☐ F ☐ S ☐ S ☐

One goal for today

_____

Today's positive affirmation

_____

_____

_____

My thoughts for today

_____

_____

_____

_____

My mood today

★ ★ ★ ★ ★ ★ ★ ★ ★ ★

Did I stay sober today?
YES ☐ NO ☐

Was today's goal accomplished?
YES ☐ NO ☐

What I am grateful for today

_____

_____

_____

What I am proud of today

_____

_____

_____

My plans for tomorrow

_____

_____

_____

_____

Date _____

M ☐ T ☐ W ☐ T ☐ F ☐ S ☐ S ☐

One goal for today

_____

_____

Today's positive affirmation

_____

_____

_____

_____

My thoughts for today

_____

_____

_____

_____

My mood today

★ ★ ★ ★ ★ ★ ★ ★ ★ ★

Did I stay sober today?
YES ☐   NO ☐

Was today's goal accomplished?
YES ☐   NO ☐

What I am grateful for today

_____

_____

_____

_____

What I am proud of today

_____

_____

_____

My plans for tomorrow

_____

_____

_____

_____

Date _____

M ☐ T ☐ W ☐ T ☐ F ☐ S ☐ S ☐

One goal for today

_____

_____

Today's positive affirmation

_____

_____

_____

_____

My thoughts for today

_____

_____

_____

_____

My mood today

★ ★ ★ ★ ★ ★ ★ ★ ★ ★

Did I stay sober today?
YES ☐   NO ☐

Was today's goal accomplished?
YES ☐   NO ☐

What I am grateful for today

_____

_____

_____

_____

What I am proud of today

_____

_____

_____

_____

My plans for tomorrow

_____

_____

_____

_____

Date _____

M ☐ T ☐ W ☐ T ☐ F ☐ S ☐ S ☐

One goal for today

_____

_____

Today's positive affirmation

_____

_____

_____

My thoughts for today

_____

_____

_____

_____

My mood today

★ ★ ★ ★ ★ ★ ★ ★ ★ ★

Did I stay sober today?
YES ☐   NO ☐

Was today's goal accomplished?
YES ☐   NO ☐

What I am grateful for today

_____

_____

_____

_____

What I am proud of today

_____

_____

_____

My plans for tomorrow

_____

_____

_____

_____

Date _____

M ☐ T ☐ W ☐ T ☐ F ☐ S ☐ S ☐

One goal for today

_____

_____

Today's positive affirmation

_____

_____

_____

_____

My thoughts for today

_____

_____

_____

_____

My mood today

★ ★ ★ ★ ★ ★ ★ ★ ★ ★

Did I stay sober today?
YES ☐   NO ☐

Was today's goal accomplished?
YES ☐   NO ☐

What I am grateful for today

_____

_____

_____

_____

What I am proud of today

_____

_____

_____

My plans for tomorrow

_____

_____

_____

_____

Date

M ☐ T ☐ W ☐ T ☐ F ☐ S ☐ S ☐

One goal for today

Today's positive affirmation

My thoughts for today

My mood today

★ ★ ★ ★ ★ ★ ★ ★ ★ ★

Did I stay sober today?
YES ☐   NO ☐

Was today's goal accomplished?
YES ☐   NO ☐

What I am grateful for today

_____

_____

_____

_____

What I am proud of today

_____

_____

_____

My plans for tomorrow

_____

_____

_____

_____

Date

M ☐ T ☐ W ☐ T ☐ F ☐ S ☐ S ☐

One goal for today

_____

_____

Today's positive affirmation

_____

_____

_____

My thoughts for today

_____

_____

_____

_____

My mood today

★ ★ ★ ★ ★ ★ ★ ★ ★ ★

Did I stay sober today?
YES ☐   NO ☐

Was today's goal accomplished?
YES ☐   NO ☐

What I am grateful for today

_____

_____

_____

_____

What I am proud of today

_____

_____

_____

My plans for tomorrow

_____

_____

_____

_____

Date _____

M ☐ T ☐ W ☐ T ☐ F ☐ S ☐ S ☐

One goal for today

_____

_____

Today's positive affirmation

_____

_____

_____

_____

My thoughts for today

_____

_____

_____

_____

_____

My mood today

★ ★ ★ ★ ★ ★ ★ ★ ★ ★

Did I stay sober today?
YES ☐   NO ☐

Was today's goal accomplished?
YES ☐   NO ☐

What I am grateful for today

_____

_____

_____

_____

What I am proud of today

_____

_____

_____

My plans for tomorrow

_____

_____

_____

_____

Date _____

M ☐ T ☐ W ☐ T ☐ F ☐ S ☐ S ☐

One goal for today

_____

_____

Today's positive affirmation

_____

_____

_____

_____

My thoughts for today

_____

_____

_____

_____

My mood today

★ ★ ★ ★ ★ ★ ★ ★ ★ ★

Did I stay sober today?
YES ☐   NO ☐
Was today's goal accomplished?
YES ☐   NO ☐
What I am grateful for today

_____

_____

_____

_____

What I am proud of today

_____

_____

_____

_____

My plans for tomorrow

_____

_____

_____

_____

Date _____

M ☐ T ☐ W ☐ T ☐ F ☐ S ☐ S ☐

One goal for today

_____

_____

Today's positive affirmation

_____

_____

_____

My thoughts for today

_____

_____

_____

_____

My mood today

★ ★ ★ ★ ★ ★ ★ ★ ★ ★

Did I stay sober today?
YES ☐   NO ☐

Was today's goal accomplished?
YES ☐   NO ☐

What I am grateful for today

_____

_____

_____

_____

What I am proud of today

_____

_____

_____

My plans for tomorrow

_____

_____

_____

_____

Date _____

M ☐ T ☐ W ☐ T ☐ F ☐ S ☐ S ☐

One goal for today

_____

_____

Today's positive affirmation

_____

_____

_____

_____

My thoughts for today

_____

_____

_____

_____

My mood today

★ ★ ★ ★ ★ ★ ★ ★ ★ ★

Did I stay sober today?
YES ☐   NO ☐

Was today's goal accomplished?
YES ☐   NO ☐

What I am grateful for today

_____

_____

_____

_____

What I am proud of today

_____

_____

_____

_____

My plans for tomorrow

_____

_____

_____

_____

Date _____

M ☐ T ☐ W ☐ T ☐ F ☐ S ☐ S ☐

One goal for today

_____

_____

Today's positive affirmation

_____

_____

_____

My thoughts for today

_____

_____

_____

_____

My mood today

★ ★ ★ ★ ★ ★ ★ ★ ★ ★

Did I stay sober today?

YES ☐   NO ☐

Was today's goal accomplished?

YES ☐   NO ☐

What I am grateful for today

_____

_____

_____

_____

What I am proud of today

_____

_____

_____

My plans for tomorrow

_____

_____

_____

_____

Date _____

M ☐ T ☐ W ☐ T ☐ F ☐ S ☐ S ☐

One goal for today

_____

_____

Today's positive affirmation

_____

_____

_____

_____

My thoughts for today

_____

_____

_____

_____

My mood today

★ ★ ★ ★ ★ ★ ★ ★ ★ ★

Did I stay sober today?
YES ☐   NO ☐
Was today's goal accomplished?
YES ☐   NO ☐
What I am grateful for today

_____

_____

_____

_____

What I am proud of today

_____

_____

_____

_____

My plans for tomorrow

_____

_____

_____

_____

Date _____

M ☐ T ☐ W ☐ T ☐ F ☐ S ☐ S ☐

One goal for today

_____

_____

Today's positive affirmation

_____

_____

_____

_____

My thoughts for today

_____

_____

_____

_____

My mood today

★ ★ ★ ★ ★ ★ ★ ★ ★ ★

Did I stay sober today?

YES ☐   NO ☐

Was today's goal accomplished?

YES ☐   NO ☐

What I am grateful for today

_____

_____

_____

What I am proud of today

_____

_____

_____

My plans for tomorrow

_____

_____

_____

Date _____

M ☐ T ☐ W ☐ T ☐ F ☐ S ☐ S ☐

One goal for today

_____

_____

Today's positive affirmation

_____

_____

_____

_____

My thoughts for today

_____

_____

_____

_____

My mood today

★ ★ ★ ★ ★ ★ ★ ★ ★ ★

Did I stay sober today?
YES ☐   NO ☐

Was today's goal accomplished?
YES ☐   NO ☐

What I am grateful for today

_____

_____

_____

_____

What I am proud of today

_____

_____

_____

My plans for tomorrow

_____

_____

_____

_____

Date

M ☐ T ☐ W ☐ T ☐ F ☐ S ☐ S ☐

One goal for today

Today's positive affirmation

My thoughts for today

My mood today

★ ★ ★ ★ ★ ★ ★ ★ ★ ★

Did I stay sober today?
YES ☐ NO ☐

Was today's goal accomplished?
YES ☐ NO ☐

What I am grateful for today

_____

_____

_____

_____

What I am proud of today

_____

_____

_____

My plans for tomorrow

_____

_____

_____

Date

M ☐ T ☐ W ☐ T ☐ F ☐ S ☐ S ☐

One goal for today

Today's positive affirmation

My thoughts for today

My mood today

★ ★ ★ ★ ★ ★ ★ ★ ★ ★

Did I stay sober today?

YES ☐   NO ☐

Was today's goal accomplished?

YES ☐   NO ☐

What I am grateful for today

_____

_____

_____

_____

What I am proud of today

_____

_____

_____

My plans for tomorrow

_____

_____

_____

_____

Date _____

M ☐ T ☐ W ☐ T ☐ F ☐ S ☐ S ☐

One goal for today

_____

_____

Today's positive affirmation

_____

_____

_____

_____

My thoughts for today

_____

_____

_____

_____

_____

My mood today

★ ★ ★ ★ ★ ★ ★ ★ ★ ★

Did I stay sober today?
YES ☐   NO ☐
Was today's goal accomplished?
YES ☐   NO ☐
What I am grateful for today

_____

_____

_____

_____

What I am proud of today

_____

_____

_____

_____

My plans for tomorrow

_____

_____

_____

_____

Made in the USA
Las Vegas, NV
15 August 2021